Burning Belly Fat or the Truth about Six Pack Abs

How to get rid of your stomach fat and develop stomach muscles in 30 minutes.

By :
Joerg Weber
http://www.welchediaet.de

Table of Content

Introduction

Chapter 1: Why a flat Stomach and a toned Figure are better for the body

Chapter 2: The fairytale about cutting fat and a flat stomach

Chapter 3: Healthy Eating

Chapter 4: Losing Weight

Chapter 5: Burning Fat

Chapter 6: Tighter and better defined stomach muscles

Chapter 7: Final Results and maintenance

Introduction

It is impossible to give an estimate about the number of people desperately looking for a way to lose the excessive fast and be fit – including being sexy and having defined abs.

As we all know, not only do we feel less attractive being overweight, but is also an unhealthy way for the body. Being overweight can lead to heart diseases, diabetes, as well as other diseases and suffering from adverse health risks.

Hence it is important to get to know methods how to lose the excessive weight and make sure that the weight stays off – for the sake not only for your health but also your self-confidence and your overall happiness.

The healthier and stronger your stomach muscles are, the better you will feel and look. Strong stomach muscles look awesome and are a good protection from having a back injury, and they help to keep a good posture. Which in turn is positive for the entire body and lets you feel more attractive and self-confident.

But there are many fairytales about the best way to accomplish this to achieve stomach muscles and the body of a celebrity. It is rather difficult to sift through all of the misleading information, appearing on the packaging of some miracle drug to lose weight and on the   instructions of the latest exercise equipment for six pack abs.

The positive matter is: You can really burn fat and at the same time develop great abs! With only a minimum of 30 minutes day! Even if you are completely out of shape and think you will never be able to do that – there is an option which will work.

Does it require a certain commitment? Yes.

Does it require a certain willingness to work on it from you? Yes.

Is it impossible to accomplish? No.

And some more positive news: If you are going to follow the program I am going to introduce to you, not only will your fat rolls be less and disappear completely at some point, but your stomach will also be ripped, sexy, and strong, and your overall health will improve.

You will feel much better, your skin and hair will look better, you will have more energy and stamina, and you will have a better immune system

I am sure you have already tries a couple of different diets and exercise programs, and that you feel discouraged by now. But if you will follow this program and will give yourself the chance to succeed you will achieve success in the long-term.

I suggest that you just read the book and take all the information to heart. Then you commit to begin a new lifestyle which will embrace everything you have learned. You will have to change fundamental things in your lifestyle. You have to eat better and exercise more - especially for your stomach area.

I am not telling you any lies, and I do not promise you that you will be slim and toned in two weeks. It is very much possible that it will take much longer. But fact is: if you never start with the program, then you will never experience the wonderful results it can bring you.

You can lose fat and bring your abs into top form along with the rest of your body. The clothes you are dying to wear will fit you again. And you can get the body you will be proud of.

Chapter 1: Why a flat Stomach and a toned Figure are better for the body

Normally people will get information about a flat stomach and losing weight because they want to look good. That is absolutely ok. We all want to look beautiful, and in today's society looking good simple means to be tight and toned because it is considered attractive.

I don't think I have to emphasize that there is a huge difference between looking good and healthy, and to look like you have starved yourself to skin and bones.

Skin and bones just does not look good, no matter what models and celebrities do. A healthy weight with a trained body and tones muscles is looking good – most people will consider this attractive.

You want to look good. That is normal and we all want to look good. Looking good has a variety of different aspects and different meanings for different people. Most people will agree if I say that a toned body looks better than a very overweight or very skinny one.

Looking good also has something to do with how you put on your make-up (if you are a female), what kind of hairstyle you have, and which clothes and accessories you are wearing. And your posture plays a big part – is it straight and conveys self-confidence, or is it curved and bent?

Do you always look well groomed and stylish? You do not have to spend crazy money for new styles and always dress like you are about to go to a party – you just have to look groomed, clean and well-coordinated. You can achieve that just as well with a white t-shirt, jeans, combed hair and a straight posture.

Think about your smile. An honest and pleasant smile is being a part of a successful appearance, as well as indication for a positive and friendly mood.

Even if you are not in perfect shape, your looks are determined as well by other factors, and that will remain the same even after you lose your weight and have toned abs.

Let's get back to your toned body. To be in shape will open doors for you. If it is fair not does not matter, but it is the truth.

People are visual creatures and a big part of the first impression someone makes is determined by how he looks. The shape you are in can make a big difference, just like the things we mentioned before like hair, cleanliness, being well groomed and your smile.

A toned and in shape body might get you more dates, or will make you more exciting for your spouse or partner.

Being trim and in shape can help you when you are looking for a job. It is a matter of fact that in some positions people who are in shape will often have an advantage when they apply for a job, or start a new career.

Is this fair? Probably not, but is in the nature of people, and you can hardly fight against it. It is much easier to get in shape and get the self-confidence which goes along with it.

There are many good reasons for a flat stomach and a toned body.

Get healthier with burning fat and toned Abs

There are a lot more reasons to lose weight and get toned abs than looking good on the beach. Your overall health will improve by exercising and losing weight.

Did you know that being trim reduced the risk of heart disease, diabetes, and that toned and strong stomach muscles also help to strengthen your back?

Let's take a look at diabetes. Type 2 diabetes is the most common diabetes type. This disease occurs when the body does not produce enough insulin, or the cells in the body do not recognize the insulin and do not use it.

Insulin is the essential component to break down Glucose (the basic fuel for the body) into energy. If your body does not use the Glucose properly, your cells will suffer from lack of energy. Over a period of time it can lead to defect of the kidneys, eyes, nerves and even the heart.

One of the biggest risk factors for Type 2 diabetes is being overweight and most of all if the weight is located around your stomach. Just to lose 15 – 20 pounds can reduce the risk of diabetes a lot.

Diabetes is a disease which needs to be taken very serious, and which can be avoided altogether, or at least delayed. If you are overweight and most of the weight is located around your stomach the risk of developing diabetes increases a lot. Three simple steps can help to prevent diabetes, and you can also get in better shape:

1. Exercise daily
2. Eat healthier
3. Lose a little weight, keep the weight steady and excercise all your muscle groups , including your stomach muscles.

Let's focus on heart disease. Do you want to do something to decrease your risk of heart disease? Then lose some weight. By losing weight you can relief your heart muscle – the most important muscle in your entire body - a little bit. It will be easier for your heart to pump blood through your body.

Your heart has to pump more blood through your body if you weigh more than you should. Instead of beating faster your heart will increase in size in order to be able to pump more blood with every beat.

The result of this can be hypertension, and the risk of having a stroke will increase. Besides higher blood pressure the heart will begin to suffer at some point in time, which may lead to congestive heart failure.

Research has shown the a waist over 35 inches for women and 39 inches for men increases the risk of heart disease, high cholesterol, and diabetes. Hence you do not just have to lose weight but also work on your waist. .

Building your abs is an added bonus in combination with reducing your waist size and with respect to health and looking good.

How strong stomach muscles can help your back.

Almost everyone will suffer from pain in their lower back at some point in their lives. Some people have this pain even all the time. A lot of times this pain is a result from the back trying to compensate for weak stomach muscles and is not caused by any injury.

Strong and trained stomach muscles will help to develop stronger torso muscles, which in turn will strengthen and support the spine. When you exercise your stomach muscles you will help to avoid a lot of back pain and problems with a slipping disc.

Many activities throughout the day will be based on your back for their movement. Just think about it – getting out of bed, opening a heavy door, carry shopping bags, pick up a child, take the dog for a walk, or check the oil in your car – all of this is extra work for your torso.

It is important to keep your stomach and torso muscles strong and healthy so your back will stay without pain.

Chapter 2: The fairytale about cutting fat and a flat stomach

I briefly mentioned this topic in the introduction: The fact that there are a lot of stubborn fairytales out there about cutting fat and rapid development of stomach muscles.

Most likely you have seen a lot of advertisement for wonder diets, wonder pills, or drinks. Or the advertising for some new exercise equipment of other technical gimmick, which will guarantee you clearly defined six pack abs within one or two weeks.

Some fairytales even tell you that you can go back to a flat stomach by eating certain nutrients, or skipping others, just like the magic disappearance and melting the fat off your body. Or that some nutrients will literally burn the fat.

The problem with all those rumors is that while they may contain some truth, there is a lot added on to them. None of those products will result in those promised results, and the reason for this is that either they are only incomplete answers to the problem how you can lose weight and train your stomach muscles, or much worse someone is trying to rip you off. Someone is trying to convince you to pay for a so-called wonder.

I know this may sound brutal, but it is a simple fact that there are a lot of fairytales and semi-truths you know and need to be careful about. In my case I would not want to sacrifice my time, energy, and money for something that will not work anyway in the end. And I do not want you to go through that either. In the end the disappointment is just too much.

I think it is much better for you if you stick to an honest and comprehensive plan, where you know it does work if you stick to it. This is much better than to eat cabbage every day, or to work with some machine to train you stomach muscles which have absolutely no effect at all.

Let's look at some of the fairytales about losing weight and stomach muscles – you will encounter them over and over again:

1. Rumor: Everything labeled „Health Food" etc. is really healthy.

Be careful with food looking especially healthy and being advertised as healthy food, yet they often skip important details like unhealthy sugar, fat, or sodium content. Some of the so-called "healthy" foods are full of chemical additives

One example is a „healthy" granola bar we see on every supermarket shelf. Granola is healthy, isn't it? Maybe. You need to read the label, the less ingredients, the better it is. Some granola bars are full of sugar and sodium. I am sorry, but too much sugar is not healthy and it will not help you to lose weight.

Another example is the so-called Light beverages. They do not contain sugar. That is really great, but the sugar substitute can be damaging to your health. Just stick to water and natural fruit juices, or tea.

2. Rumor: A crash diet can help you losing weight for good

If someone promises you a miracle within a couple days and will animate you to eat a very imbalanced you can call it a crash diet. It can very well be that you will lose weight, but it will be very difficult to keep the weight off afterwards – except you intend to eat imbalanced meals for the rest of your life. This would not be healthy, and if you are not healthy then it does not really matter how fit you are.

Crash diets result in a rapid weight loss, which is impossible to maintain in the long term. In addition to that they are so unhealthy that they may really damage your health. It is much smarter to learn how to eat right. If you accomplish that you will be able to lose weight and keep it off.

3. Rumor: There are certain foods that will make you lose weight

This would be fabulous – but it is not true. There is no food which will burn fat or help you lose pounds. Some foods can accelerate the metabolism for a short period of time (like green tea), but you cannot really lose weight with them

4. Rumor: Fat burning pills are effective

There are no pills you can take and you will burn fat. Every dietary supplement which suppresses your appetite contains certain risk.

5. Rumor: If it is labeled natural it will be efficient and you can take it without a doubt.

Not necessarily. There are so many supplements with „natural "of „organic"contents on the market, which does not mean that they are either safe or effective. Do you know about Ephedra? ?

It is an organic ingredient, which claims to help you lose weight, but at the same time there is a risk of serious side effects and can cause serious health problems, which can even cause death. Just because the product label states it does not contain Ephedra, does not mean automatically it will not be dangerous. Neither does it mean that it will help to burn fat or help develop stomach muscles.

6. Rumor: A lot of stomach exercises and sit-ups or using exercise equipment – the best method to get defined stomach muscles.

I will not tell you to do stomach exercises – but you cannot rely entirely on sit-ups or a stomach exercise equipment to trim your waist and sculpt your stomach. You have to use a combination of the right exercise and right nutrition. There is no other way.

Most of the time stomach exercise equipment is just a waste of money. You can do the exact same exercises without a piece of equipment. These are just tricks to make you believe that you will get the six pack abs within a short period of time if you use it daily. There is much more to it to get the perfect body. Don't throw your money out of the window.

7. Rumor: Do not lift weights; it will make you look bigger

Strength workout and weight lifting builds muscles, and more muscles burn more calories. Building muscles will help with the weight loss. Two to three times strength workout is ideal and will not make your muscles look bulky. It will help you lose weight and will make you look much more attractive.

Lifting weights does not have to be severe labor in order to benefit from it. Even working with some light weights or a medicine ball will help you build muscles.

8. Rumor: To lose weight you will have to do a lot of Aerobics

It is true that you need to do Aerobics to stay healthy, to lose weight easier and to burn fat, but it does not need to be the only ways you exercise you need to do to burn fat and build your stomach muscles. And much less you need to do aerobics until you are exhausted and pass out. Instead you should mix aerobics with strength workout and stretching, which is the best way to burn fat and build muscles.

9. Rumor: Carbs are bad

This just is not true. You need carbs in your diet, but you have to pay attention to eat the right carbs. Single carbs like you will find in white bread are not healthy. Complex carbs like the ones in multi grain bread will even help you to burn fat.

10. Rumor: You should cut fat from your diet completely

This not true either. A certain amount of fat (the right kind of fat) is necessary for your health and does not prevent losing weight or cutting fat. .

11. Rumor: To lose weight quickly is the best way

No. It is unhealthy to lose weight too quick. And it is nearly impossible to maintain a rapid weight loss in the long-term. It is much better to lose continuously and slow. Even if you would like to slim down in a few days or weeks – it is simply not realistic to achieve great results like that.

Another reason not to lose fat so quick is that your skin will need time to tighten. Especially people who want to lose a lot of weight will have a lot of skin-folds. To prevent that you should settle for a steady weight loss (not more than 2 pounds a week). This way, your skin can tighten better with the rest of the body while you get toned.

12. Rumor: You can get a six pack abs in „ five easy steps"(or three or seven etc.)

You will get a flat stomach with muscles through hard work and a combination of different exercises with a healthy and low fat diet. To follow "five easy steps" will not get you a flat stomach and much less six pack abs. I do not want to discourage youth all, you can get a great stomach with a lot of toned muscles. But it takes a lot more work than a few exercises.

13. Rumor: Targeted workout of a certain spot will be effective!

If you try to burn fat at a certain spot with specific exercises it will not be successful. Key to a flat stomach or to a well-defined other area of your body is to stimulate your metabolism. This way it will cut the unnecessary fat around your waist and other areas of your body. Once the fat is gone and your muscles are toned they will show. This is the way it works.

14. Rumor: When exercising quantity is better than quality

To exercise your stomach is not everything. Some people believe that they should do 100 routines of jackknives, even if they do it halfheartedly. This is not true. It is much better to do less or different exercises the right way and slower, even if you can only do less of them. In the long-term this will be much more effective.

You will find these fairytales all the time in the internet and in newspapers. Even in the supermarket or the pharmacy you will find odds and ends of food and weight loss products which are advertised to be healthy and helpful in losing weight

Countless TV spots will try to motivate you to buy another one of the brand new exercise equipment for a flat stomach, and you will be promised to have a flat sexy stomach in absolutely no time. In another spot they will try to sell you a diet drink, consisting of cabbage juice and yoghurt. The promise is that pounds will melt like the snow in the spring sun and you will look like a model

Of course we all do want to believe these lies. We want to believe that the fat around our waist will disappear after 200 sit ups per day, and leave behind a stomach were everyone will be jealous. But unfortunately the fairytales and rumors are exactly that - fairytales and rumors.

Time to get back to reality, which means: Burning far, losing weight and a sexy, flat stomach are the results of a combination of different things – if want to call it that way, it is an attack from different angles. You will need a lot of commitment and dedication.

Don't let this deter yourself. You can do it. Whether you want to lose 10 pounds because you have a little beer belly or 100 pounds and know very well that this will be hard work to train your stomach muscles so you can show them off – You can do it.

Fairytales and lies aim for one thing only – to sell you something. Instead of being misled try to use your time, energy and hard earned money to do something much more worthwhile: to develop healthy eating habits, to learn the right kind of exercise which will burn fat and speed up your metabolism. The goal is to move your body in a way that not only your stomach muscles, but also all the other muscles will be strengthened, trained and toned.

Does this happen overnight? In one week? In two weeks? No. It will take time. You might have to wait a couple weeks to start seeing results. End it will take even longer to see the final goal you are trying to reach.

Everything depends on the condition you are in when you start. But if you eat right and sacrifice half an hour every day to train - you will be able to succeed!

Just be very conscious that the best and really the only right way to it are to start the *right* way. That means to eat right and move your body.

The remainder of this book will discuss how to develop healthy eating habits, to lose weight at a healthy pace, burning fat and to sculpt a trim and flat stomach. You will learn a lot, and when you are through you will be armed to tackle the extra weight and a flabby stomach.

If you ask yourself if you can try a certain food, a trick or a piece of exercise equipment while you are working according to the plan I am going to introduce in the book, the answer will certainly be: yes , of course , if you insist on it. But please be careful with any kind of pills and nutritional supplements. Don't throw your money out of the window; it does not matter whether it is for pills, supplements or an equipment to exercise your stomach muscles.

Most likely those methods will not help at all and might even cause damage. If you insist on spending money, you should buy a set of dumbbells or a light medicine ball. Thise are helpful and effective.

Chapter 3: Healthy Eating

I should not really have to tell you that you should only eat healthy foods. This is not rocket science. Ever since you have been a child you have heard – eat your vegetables, don't eat too much ice-cream, and so many chips and French fries, it's better to eat lean meat, bla , bla , bla.

It is just a fact, that many of us like the „bad" stuff and don't eat enough of the „good" stuff. The world has become much faster and busier. Everything seems to be done fast frozen, salted, sugared and packaged – we got used to eat this way.

This is not healthy and for sure not good for your waist or to make your stomach muscles appear, which is hidden under a flabby layer of fat. If you are not getting rid of the fat, you will never see those muscles.

It does not matter how many stomach exercises you do, or how many lengths you swim; burning fat and a sexy stomach start with healthy eating, There is no way around it – if you have not been eating healthy until now, you need to start.

Besides the fact that you will get a beautiful body, healthy eating also means you will feel better, have more energy, a better mood and will have a better immune system. To eat healthy does wonders for you.

How eating right will give you more energy

Our bodies get their energy they use to accomplish all the tasks we want to do and expect from them from the food we eat. You know we will die without eating because out bodies cannot produce energy themselves. Food is necessary.

The body transforms food into Glucose (blood sugar) and produces energy. Carbs are the easiest to convert to energy; hence they are to most important ingredient to keep our energy at a constant level.

The only problem is to know which carbs are good for you and create a constant energy level, and which ones are not so healthy and will only spike the energy level for a short period of time in order to let it plunge so you will feel tired and lazy.

Simple carbs like sugar and the ones you find in white bread etc. Can be converted to energy very quickly. As a result you will dope yourself. Then the blood sugar- and energy level will drop rapidly and will cause an effect where you will have a hard time to move around.

Complex Carbs like the ones in whole grain bread will give your body energy much slower, but this energy will last much longer. Like this you will create a constant energy flow throughout the day and will feel much better and stronger.

Taking in complex cards will also help to avoid the energy slump in the afternoon from which many of us suffer.

Instead you will have plenty of energy from morning until night time

In order to keep a higher energy level without constant ups and downs it is best to take in a lot of complex carbs like protein (which your body will also convert to energy) and low fat foods. Do not eat too many simple carbs.

Following a list of the most important foods with complex carbs:
- Whole Grain Pasta
- Brown Rice
- Grain like Barley, Wheat and Oats
- Whole Grain Bread (wheat, oats, bran, etc.)
- Whole Grain Cereal (pay attention to sugar content)
- Oatmeal
- Sweet Potatoes
- Peas, Beans , and other Legumes

And following a list with foods you should avoid because they   contain   simple   carbs:

- Processed sugar
- White Bread, Buns
- Sweets
- Chocolate
- Deserts
- Sweet Snacks
- Sugar coated grain

Remarks: some fruits are labeled as simple carbs because they have high fruit sugar content. Which means they quickly spike the energy levle, which will decrease soon thereafter. But the fruit is still very good for the body and plays a vital part in burning fat and losing weight. Eat fruits!

Breakfast and lunch should be your most important meals of the day, your diner should be rather small - before you go to sleep you won't need a lot of calories or energy. You can also eat two smaller snacks during the day so your energy level won't drop. However, do pay attention not to get too many calories.

As for snack which taste good and are low in fat and calories you could eat something like yoghurt mixes with granola (unsweetened), a hand full almonds, or a chicken sandwich with whole grain bread and low fat mayonnaise.

While you are working to lose weight and burn fat you still need to eat right. If you do not fuel your body with energy you will not feel like exercising. Exercising is a very important part of burning fat and building muscles. The right nutrition will provide more energy on a constant level because your body receives the proper fuel - fuel which is burnt constantly.

If we talk about energy we mean carbs most the time, but also alcohol, protein, and fats are converted into energy by the body as well. Alcohol burns very quickly, the body will always use it first; reason being is that it cannot store any energy coming from alcohol. Trying to lose weight you should consume little alcohol, if at all, because it will prevent your body from using carbs, protein and fat.

Protein will be converted into energy by your body. It is important to get enough protein to supply your body with the building blocks for muscles, cells, and energy

Fat is the last component the body will burn as fuel. You should not consume too much fat, especially if you are already overweight. If you are eating right and watch how many calories you eat will help your body to burn stored fat cells and to burn what has been deposited on your stomach and your waistline.

Why do you need fat in your nutrition

Even if you are just in the process to lose fat, you still have to take in fat every day. Why?
- Fat is protection for vital organs in your body
- Fat keeps skin and nails healthy
- Fat keeps your hair healthy (and on your head)
- Fat helps with digestion
- Fat helps the body to absorb vitamin A, D, E, and K
- Fat helps to keep the cell membranes functional

Even though we do need a certain amount of fat in our nutrition, most of us will still take in way to much every day. Fat in small portions is ok. How many grams of fat do you need each day?
In general you can follow this calculation:

If you take in 1200 calories per day, you should consume about 40 grams of fat. If you eat 1500 calories per day, you will need about 50 grams of fat. At 2000 calories you will already need 65 grams of fat. How much fat is in your food is easy to read on the product labels and in nutrition guidelines.

Which fats are good and which are bad?

There is another factor you need to pay attention to before you avoid fat altogether or eat too much of it. Some are better for us than others. If you are consuming fat, then it should be the "healthy" ones. You should always stay away from the "unhealthy" fat. „Good Fats" are the ones with mono- and poly-unsaturated fatty acids.

Mono unsaturated fatty acids will lower cholesterol and can also be helpful sometimes to fight body fat. Still this does not mean you should consume too many of them, it simple states that they can be helpful. Nuts, Avocados, Olive oil, and Rapeseed oil contain mono saturated fatty acids.

Poly unsaturated fatty acids can help to lower cholesterol as well. They contain lot of Omega-3 fatty acids, which can prevent heart disease. Fish oil, Corn oil, Canola oil, Soy oil, Sunflower Seed oil and Safflower oil contain poly unsaturated fatty acids.

You should read all the labels and stick to it. Bad Fats are for example saturated fatty acids and trans fat.

Saturated fatty acids will raise your cholesterol level and the risk for heart disease. Meat, dairy products, eggs and some seafood contain saturated fat, just like coconut fat, palm oil and palm kernel oil.

Trans fats are a sort of artificial fat you will find in many commercially packaged foods and fast food, as well as in Margarine and plant oils. Trans fats are unhealthy because they increase the risk of heart disease and the cholesterol level.

Do not try to eliminate fat complete from your diet, but bear in mind that you are reading this book because you have consumed to much fat all along.

What may appear normal is most likely much too much, and you can only lose weight and get those stomach muscles if you are going to get rid of the stored fat. You can eat fat, just becarfeul whatyou eat.

Protein – Building blocks for strong stomach muscles

Sometimes you are told to eat a lot of protein in order to get those perfect abs. While protein is of course important and necessary as building block for your stomach muscles, besides for about everything else in your stomach as well, it is never a good idea to exaggerate

A healthy, fat- and calorie reduced diet with enough protein does not just help to build stomach muscles, but generally aides building muscles. In addition it is helping to keep your cells, bones, hair, and nails healthy.

You do not have to buy some of this expensive protein powder in order to have enough protein in your diet. Just stick to the following simple steps and this will be more than   enough:

- Eat lean meat, like chicken (without the skin) and any other poultry, pork tenderloin, and lean beef.
- Eat more fish. Fish and seafood are excellent sources for protein, and most of the time low in fat. Another added benefit is Omega-3 fatty acids, which are excellent for your heart.
- Beans and nuts contain a lot of protein. In turn nuts can also be very fatty. Pay attention to the size of the portion – best just a handful (approx. 7 ounces)
- Low-fat dairy products contain protein. You should eat low-fat yoghurt, milk and cheese. This is also an excellent source for calcium.
- Egg whites contain protein and little fat and are great for losing weight and a source for calcium.
- Multi grain bread and other multi grain products contain protein as well.

Most of the people eat enough protein each day to build muscle. It means that you do not need extra protein even with intensive work outs, as long as you pay attention and eat healthy.

The Food Pyramid – still very helpful

Most likely you have heard about the food pyramid before. Perhaps you learned about it in school. Everything we like to eat was in the very tip of the pyramid, or was missing completely (where for example was the chocolate cake?).

Maybe this looks like a very old-fashioned way to select your food, but it is still a very helpful guideline. On the bottom you will find the grains, after that fruit and vegetables, followed by dairy products and protein, last but not least on the tip of it fat, oils, and sweets (and that is where the chocolate cake is hiding!)

It is recommended to eat six to eleven servings of grain (bread, cornflakes, pasta, rice), three to five servings of vegetables and two to four servings of fruit, two to three servings each of dairy and proteins, but only a little bit of fat and oil.

This is not too much, even for someone trying to lose weight. But we need to keep in mind that the recommended servings are much smaller than the portions we normally eat. You also have to pay attention which foods you are eating, even if they are part of the pyramid.

The food pyramid shows us what our body needs in order to function properly and to stay healthy. It is a guideline about the amount we should eat from each type of food. And that is the reason why it is a good base for a healthy diet; again, it should not be the only guideline we use.

Your idea of portion size is most likely wrong

During the course of many years we were lead to believe that a portion of food is much larger than it should be. Our picture of portions has been skewed, based on the oversized portions in restaurants. And it is one of the reasons for weight gain. In order to tackle this problem you need to know how big a serving should be:

Bread

1 slice – about half the size of a CD cover
2 ½ - 6 inch pancakes
½ a sausage or bun

Rice and Pasta

7 ounces pasta, spaghetti, macaroni, or rice

Vegetables

1 small baked potato or 4.5 fl. ounces mashed potatoes
3.5 ounces peas or corn
7 ounces pumpkin
3.5 ounces beans or lentil
7 ounces raw vegetables or salad

Fruit

1 small apple, or 3.5 ounces unsweetened apple sauce
12-15 Grapes
7 ounces Melon
7 ounces Raspberries
2 small plums
1 medium size Orange

Dairy

8.4 fl. ounces Milk
8.4 fl. ounces Soy Milk
8.4 fl. ounces yoghurt
1.4 – 2.0 ounces Cheese

Meat, poultry, and Tofu

1 portion is about the size of a playing card

Fish

1 portion is about the size of a check book

Oil
One portion is about a tea spoon

Salad Dressing
One portion is two tea spoons

Nuts
One portion is about 0.7 ounces

This is not a complete list at all; you could very well fill an entire book about portion size for any kind of food.

However, it is sufficient that you know the above. You were probably quite surprised about some of the serving sizes. Maybe now you start to blame yourself because you have been eating portions which were way too big and did not think anything of it. If you want to be successful in losing weight you should start to pay attention to the portions you eat.

What you should avoid

Now you know that you should stay away from those huge ice-cream sundaes and an entire fried chicken, but you should also know that you need to avoid the following:
- Fatty meat and poultryfettiges Fleisch und Geflügel
- Food with a high fat content Nahrungsmittel mit hohem Fettgehalt

Don't by marbeled meats, stick to lean filets. And

whenever possible try to buy reduced fat or fat free versions of the food you usually buy. Believe me the fat your body needs you will be able to get somewhere else

Chapter 4: Losing Weight

To burn fat, lose weight, and build your stomach muscles – that is your goal. It is really a three part mission in order to improve your body, your health, and your life. Each of those three will be most effective if you tackle the other two at the same time. It is much easier to master one part if you work on the other two at the same time.

Losing weight is not as easy as we would like it to be. It does require commitment and determination. You have to want it so much, that you are willing to put it ahead of the things you normally like to do, or eat. Your improved health, elevated self-confidence as you will start to look better, should make it well worth the effort.

In order to lose weight you have to feed your body less fuel than it needs. This will force your body to use the fuel it already has in form of fat. To lose weight means to feed you with fewer calories and less fat.

Try some endurance workout or other exercises for your stomach area, and it will help you to lose weight faster, burn fat more effectively and build those stomach muscles you so want to have.

Experts recommend losing continuously and no more than 2 pounds per week in order to lose weight in a way that you will be able to maintain it in the long-term. Even though it may not seem much; it will pay off in the long run and is much healthier for your body.

Losing weight slow and steady is also a much better way if you have to lose a lot of weight and are afraid you might end up with big skinfolds. If you are losing weight slowly your skin is much better able to gain back some of the elasticity and tighten up in the process. The skinfolds will be reduced to a bearable amount.

When you are losing weight slowly you will also be sure that your body does burn fat and does not lose muscle. Another bonus is that none of your other organs will suffer with the sudden and rapid weight loss.

If you are losing weight too fast it can lead to losing important minerals from your body and you will experience fatigue, cramps and nausea. You can even suffer from hair loss. But by far the worst is that your body will believe that it is starving and will then consequentially stop to fuel your metabolism and try to defend the energy it has stored as much as possible.

How to lose weight

The basic principle of losing weight is to create a calorie deficit, which means your calorie intake will be less than what your body needs. As previously mentioned you can do this with the following steps:

First you determine how many calories you need to eat. You can find the calories for most of the foods or drinks easily in the internet. Product information and labels also inform you about the calories.

Don't skip anything when you calculate the calories! Eat meals you prepare yourself and look at the individual ingredients and amounts to see how the calories are being added up.

Pay attention to all the values for at least a week, longer however is even better. This way you will find out how many calories as being added up with the regular food and drinks you take in, and also see what you need to skip. The amount of calories does not have to add up to the exact amount, but try to get as close as possible.

Write down the exact amount of calories you consume during this phase. You need to write down everything you eat - even cookies and chewing gum. Just use a little notebook. Follow this for at least one week; don't even skip the teaspoon of sugar you may put on your cornflakes or in your coffee.

You will realize exactly where you need to cut down. If you can consume 500 calories less each day you will lose about one pound per week. If you exercise you will burn additional calories.

If you eat 500 calories less per day and lose another 250 by exercising, you will cut 5.250 calories per week, or about two pounds. It is not that difficult, you just have to do it. .

Simple ways to reduce your caloric intake: don't put sugar in your coffee, for your afternoon snack replace sweets and chocolate with fruit or vegetables, or even better do not eat sweets except one desert a week.

Another easy change: put mustard on your sandwich instead of mayonnaise; eat clear soups instead of creamy ones, etc. If you examine your eating habits in detail you will find additional options where you can reduce calories. But you will not have the feeling that you are really missing out on anything by switching to smaller portions.

Look back at chapter three: healthy nutrition, serving sizes and healthier foods with less fat and calories. Take another look at the food pyramid. This will help you to prepare healthy meals with a lot of nutritional value, but without a lot of fat and calories, which will only add to your waistline.

Plan your meals and snacks ahead of time. Don't wait until you are starving and can wharf down an entire bag of chips just to fill up your stomach. Take the time to plan what you would like to eat.

There are a lot of great cookbooks out there for people who are looking to lose weight, with a lot of delicious recipes, which are easy to prepare, have little calories and fat, but still taste great. You can also find a lot of recipes on the internet for every taste, and very suitable for anyone trying to eat healthy and well while losing weight. .

Try to eat foods which are high in fiber. Fiber will make you feel full faster and longer. There are plenty of foods, which are high in fiber and low in calories, such as:

- Whole grain products (without added sugar) Vollkorngetreideprodukte (ohne Zuckerzusatz)
- While grain bread and pasta
- Chick peas
- Any fresh fruit ansd vegetables

Drink water – a lot of water! Water is essential for your health, and it helps to prevent bloating. If you drink a lot of water your bodies is able to burn fat faster and get rid of toxins.

Without a plan you will fail

If you are trying to lose weight it does not help if you are not setting goals for yourself. Setting goals is exactly the right tool in order to turn you efforts to lose weight into a success.

As almost everyone knows, it is generally impossible to get to where you want to be without a plan how to get there, don't you agree? And exactly this is the point when you are setting your goals. Set yourself a final goal and several steps how you want to get there, this will be the way to your dream body.

The problem is that not everyone knows how to set effective goals to reach your final goal. It is not enough to tell yourself "I will lose 40 pounds and will have six pack abs." You need to have a very specific goal and detailed intermediate goals to reach on your way to your six pack abs.

For example, your goal could look like this:

Final Goal: to lose 40 pounds in 25 weeks. To exercise my stomach muscles so I can show them off, to exercise so that the rest of my body is tight and toned, reduce cellulite on my thighs to wear skinny jeans, without a muffin top.

Those goals are setting the bar very high, but they are very specific at the same time. You know exactly what you want to reach. However, you now have to define intermediate goals , single small steps, which are going to keep you motivated after you reach them, and will encourage you to reach the next goal.

You can set your intermediate goals in a very short time frame in order to keep motivating yourself after you reach each individual goal and continue to fight for what you want. Of course you can also spread them further apart, and this could look like that:

Goal after the first month: Lose 6 pounds by reducing daily calories by 500 – 750. Exercise 30 minutes every day (a combination of aerobics and exercises for your stomach muscles), in order to burn additional 150 – 250 calories each day. To try new recipes which are low calorie and low fat.

Goal after the second month: Lose an additional 6 pounds so that the overall weight loss is 12 pounds. Continue the plan to eat less and excercise. Try to aim for a higher exercise goal and start interval training. Try to intensive exercising and burn more calories and fat so your overall wieght loss will accelerated. Your clothes will fit pretty loosely by now !

This is how you set your goals. Some people prefer to set the individual goals closer together, perhaps every week or every other week. That is quite alright. Your individual goals should be a challenge, but yet you should be able to reach them in order to keep your motivation level high. If you set your individual goals too high it is easy to get discouraged and to give up.

Pay attention that your final goal is realistic. If you dream of looking like a movie star in the end , then you really need to get a reality check. Not that it is impossible, but movie stars do have some plastic surgery done in order to correct all the little flaws. They have personal trainers monitoring their exercise program - sometimes several hours per day. And they live in a world where black coffee and a cigarette may pass for a meal (This is really not a good way to lose weight)

A lot of times you can read that most of your favorite actresses do not consume more than 900 calories per day in order to stay really skinny and look the way we think they should look. For one this is very hard to accomplish, and also not a very good method to lose weight in the long run, and keep it off as well.

Believe me, by following this program you will look fabulous when you have reached your goal. But still you have to be reasonable. Be realistic and keep reminding yourself that the most important thing is still to be happy and healthy, not just to have a trimmed and toned body and killer abs.

Don't be afraid to set individual goals and an overall goal. The individual goals are a great motivation and help you to accomplish what you really want. To set a goal for yourself is always a good method to achieve something, not only when it comes to shedding pounds, but for any goal in your life. .

Aids and support when losing weight

If you are on the track of losing weight some aides can be very helpful to keep motivated and on the right track. I keep imagining a "motivation tool chest" you carry around constantly. This way you are not going to lose sight over your progress, but will also be encouraged in case your motivation drops.

This „tool chest" does not need to be a real chest, but you can for example put your aides for losing weight in a drawer or a box – this is entirely up to you.

Trying to lose weight you will have different aides to choose from. You can use all of them, or just select a few. Either is ok, but for most of the people it is better, and easier to have several different options. You can choose the following diet aides:

A diet diary – this is one of the basics when you start, but also during losing weight and after you accomplish your goal (and would like to maintain the weight), and it will help you to stay motivated.
You can choose a simple note pad or a high end dairy you bought in a store. Or try to keep your diet diary on your computer or even online.

This diet diary will also help you to stay focused about the things you eat, how you feel before and after a meal, the location , time, place and other information to help you identify the reason and motives about your eating habit, as well as to document your progress.

For some people the diet dairy is a great tool to identify right away when you develop bad eating habits, and can aid to stop them immediately.

Pictures – how about some photos of you in the tool chest? Try to take pictures of you along the way and put them in the chest, this will show you the progress you make. It will encourage and motivate you. To pin them on your fridge might also be a good idea.

Quotes and proverbs – some people may think this is really something silly, but for many people it can do miracles. Almost everybody repeats certain things to encourage himself. Why not put up your favorite quotes and proverbs citing motivation and faith in you, health, self-confidence, etc. where you can see them every day as motivation?

Rewards – no „motivation tool chest „ is complete without a reward for the individual goals and the final goal. Those can be tangible things you put aside to reward yourself, or maybe even just a plain and simple thought about something to do when you are crossing the finish line – perhaps a manicure, buy new cross trainers you always wanted to have, tickets to a Baseball game or a concert you wanted to see for such a long time.

An exercise diary – An exercise diary can also be a part of your diet diary; however you might easily get confused. It is better to have a second diary where you document your routines, how long the last, how you feel before and after, and of course the visible results.

This diary will help you to see which of the exercises are working well, when, and how you should do them. You will see much quicker if you should make some changes to your routine.

Another „aid" you need is support. You can't fit a group of supporters in the tool chest, yet it can have an enormous impact on losing weight and exercising. Not everyone likes to engage others in the project weight loss, but a lot of people do it because it helps them along.

Try to select some friends for this support. They will help you to stay on course, give you a subtle hint, if you are drifting away from the plan, and encourage and motivate you if things do not go exactly according to plan.

All you need are people on whose support you can rely on. Folks who just smile at you and have a negative attitude can't help you.

Sometimes is just works out great to team up with another person who is also losing weight and exercises – you can do it together while you encourage and motivate each other. Just like in many other situations in life it is much easier to achieve your goals together with a friend or a likeminded group as this will create positive support, ideas, and motivation.

Chapter 5: Burning Fat

One of the reasons why you are reading this book is obviously that you are hoping to learn how you can get rid of excessive weight which you are lugging around on certain parts of your body. You already know by now that you have to burn it somehow, either by eating less so that your body is forced to turn the fat into energy, or by losing it with exercising, where the fat will also be transformed into energy.

Before we continue, there are some things about fat and its use by our body. This knowledge will help you to do anything you can for your body to use the excess fat. It is now about time that we talk about your metabolism, what fat actually is, how the body uses it, and of course how we can get our body to use more of it. Besides this we will discuss other important topics about burning fat as well.

Why is the metabolism so important?

Metabolism is a word you will hear over and over again in connection with diet and losing weight. You can hear people complaining about their slow metabolism, and cite this as the reason why they are not losing weight. But what exactly is metabolism?

To put it into simple terms, the metabolism is the amount of energy (in form of calories) which the body uses to keep functioning. Everything you do – walk, sleep, read, surf the internet, work.... your body will burn calories with everything you do. Your metabolism is based on the fact how fast and efficient you can burn those calories (stored energy).

The metabolism is influenced mainly by how much fat and how many muscles your body has. The more muscles you have, the more calories you will need to function. Muscles need more calories than fat.

People with a small percentage of body fat and a higher percentage of muscles have a faster metabolism than the ones with less muscles and more fat.

They are overweight and out of shape, no you do not have to panic. If you start with the program to lose weight and build muscles your metabolism with increase and you will burn fat! The more fat you burn and the more muscles you built your metabolism will increase. And so on and so forth.

Your metabolism, even if he is slow and maybe your enemy right now; you will be able to turn him into one of your best friends. It is simply done by eating healthy, low fat and low calorie every day and of course with the right amount of exercise.

What is fat and how can it be converted to energy?

The fat which our bodies carry around with themselves was not really produced by them. The amount of fat cells (also called Adipocytes) is given to you at birth. These are the cells with the clear task to store fat.

The body does not produce any new fat cells, it only fills them - they are the storage units for energy (energy in form of fat). The way how fat reaches those cells is actually pretty straight forward.

You eat something and your body breaks the food down into smaller parts – fat, protein, Carbs, etc. Depending how much energy your body needs it will use the fat quickly, or it will store it for later use.

Some of the stored fat is even good for your body, no matter if you want to believe it or not, because it helps to protect your internal organs and aides the proper function of bodily systems.

But if you store more fat then the body needs for energy, protection, or to function well, you will store it on your hips, your buttocks, or other parts where it will look ugly. Our goal is that the body will use the fat it originally stored for later on.

As soon as the body will need energy and has to access the fat cells in order to use the deposited fat it creates a chemical process. This process transforms the fat in the fat cells into fatty acids, which the muscles will use as energy.

This is a rather complicated process (But which body function isn't complicated?), whereas for us the only important thing is that the fat will be taken from the fat cells. Through blood circulation it will be transported to the place where it is needed as fuel.

Why can't you burn fat in just one spot?

Most likely you have heard about targeted weight loss at one of the problem zones – your waist, perhaps your buttocks, or on your thighs. There is a lot of good advertising out there trying to convince you that all it takes is to focus on that certain area where you want to lose weight and this is where the fat will be burned.

We are really sorry, but it does not work this way.

Burning and building fat always involves the entire body. If fat is used from the fat cells where it is stored, it will be taken from all the cells in your body, not only from one area. It does not matter how determined you exercise the specific area, or how you are trying to convince your body in any other way to take fat only from this very place: fat is always burned from your entire body.

As already said, you are born with a certain amount of fat cells. It is correct that they may be more in certain areas of your body. And as soon as your body starts to burn fat they will lose whatever they have stored. Not just some, but all of them. You will lose fat everywhere in your body and not only in the location you believe to be too fat.

The result: Your whole body will be tighter. It could very well be that you still have too much mass in some places, but that's genetics. If you are losing weight all around and exercise the rest, so that you will look trim and toned you will look just fabulous!

How you burn fat in 30 minutes per day

Now let's get to the exciting part. You are eating less, and what you are eating is healthy, right? You stick to a new and healthy diet, where you consume less fat and calories, but still receive the proper nutrition you need to stay strong and healthy. Now it is about time to burn fat!

The only want to burn fat is to work it off. This means you will have to move. If you prefer to sit on the couch in front of the TV all night you won't really like this part so much. But, believe me; you will feel so much better once you begin to exercise. You will feel better, healthier and have more energy. And of course at some point you will look better!

Your exercise to burn fat will alternate with specific exercises for your torso muscles. You should exercise 30 minutes every day, seven days per week.

In order to burn fat you have to start with endurance training, at least every other day. It is excellent for your heart and lung, and every other part of your body. Your metabolism will speed up and your body will have to use stored energy to move and support the faster metabolism.

Endurance workout is most effective when you alternate between easy, medium and intensive sets. During intensive sets the heart will be at approximately 75% - 85% of its maximum frequency. You will feel much challenged during the intensive routine. You will still be able to talk but you will not have enough breath for an ongoing conversation. Intensive workout does help a lot when you are trying to burn fat. However, you should not do it every time you exercise. Once a weak is enough.

You should exercise with intermediate routines about once or twice a week. This kind of exercise will challenge your heart at approximately 60% - 70% of its heart frequency. You will be able to carry a conversation, even though it might be more strenuous than when you are sitting on the couch and talk to someone. Even an intermediate workout is still very effective to burn fat.

And last but not least, you need light endurance workout for a weekly balance. These routines are more pleasant than the intermediate or intensive ones, but they can still be effective in your fight against too many calories and too much fat.

With the light endurance workout your heart will be challenged about 50% - 55% of its maximum frequency. You should use this workout once a week.

Your endurance workout schedule could look like this:

1st Week:
Monday: intermediate endurance workout
Wednesday: intensive training
Friday: light endurance workout

2nd Week:
Sunday: intermediate endurance workout
Tuesday: intensive training
Thursday: light endurance training
Sunday: intermediate endurance workout

On the days where you don't schedule endurance workout you will do your stomach and torso muscles exercises. Combined with a healthy, low fat and low calorie diet you will look leaner and more toned.

What kind of exercise is right for intensive training?

In general you can do any exercise as intensive workout—walking , bicycling , jogging, running, swimming, dancing, kickboxing – all of this you can do very intense. Intensive workout does not necessarily be the same for you as for someone else, as we all are individuals with a very different condition. If you are starting to sweat a lot and you have a hard time carrying a conversation with someone, then you can call it intensive training.

You will not need any kind of special gear for intensive training. You can get some dancing or aerobic CD's and excercise at home. If you like to ride bike, just do it more intense. Or walk a little faster than you normally would, start to jog. You should keep the intensive pace for about half an hour. If you can't do the entire 30 minutes in the beginning just work your way up to it. Give your very best.

Intermediate endurance workout?

You can do the same exercises with the intermediate endurance workout just at a more moderate pace. Again you do not need any special gear. During the intermediate endurance workout you will breathe heavier, sweat and feel challenged, but you can still carry a conversation. If this is not enough for you, you can easily switch to intensive workout for a couple minutes. This will you will burn some extra calories and fat. A good Pilates or Yoga DVD, or a light Aerobic CD will be sufficient for the intermediate training.

And the light endurance workout?

During the light endurance workout you will give your body a break to recover from the activities of the past couple days. You are still exercising and this is important. Even light endurance workout will burn fat, especially if you have been exercising according to your plan on all the previous days.

Light endurance workout can consist of walking, a long but slow bicycle ride, a little bit of yoga, a couple of laps in the pool, yard work, walking with the dog, washing the car (of course manually, not the car wash) or any kind of lighter activities where your body will be in motion and your heart beats a little faster than normal.

Now that you understand the difference between the various forms of endurance workout and know how you should change out the routines you will have to learn another very important part to burn fat: You have to be very consistent.

If you are not consistent there is no way you will achieve the desired result. To exercise continuously means seven days a week, half an hour a day. This is the only way for your body to burn fat effective. You will carry oxygen in every cell in of the body, which in turn will help the cells to burn fat faster.

The fatty acids in your body will be ready to be used as fuel much faster as your bloodstream will improve with consistent exercise, and your body can produce energy much more efficient from this fuel.

Endurance workout is much better outdoors, if the weather is nice enough. If you live in a place with a very cold winter, or incredibly hot summers, it would be ideal to get an exercise machine for indoors. You can use it on days where you cannot exercise outdoors.

One alternative would be a good fitness center. You can get workout guides tailored individually according to your fitness level, you will have access to all the equipment you need and there are often special group sessions you can participate in.

Interval Training: A secret weapon

Maybe you have heard about interval workout before. Previously I suggested that to add to your intermediate endurance training, without calling it interval training.

Interval workout is a workout where you intensify your workout after a certain period of time, even if the phase only lasts one or two minutes. Your body shifts into a much higher gear and it will be much easier to burn calories and fat

Interval workout is very simple – intensify your motion. Walk or bike faster, choose a path leading uphill. Find a way to exercise more intense, faster, more challenging or harder.

Ideally you will start out normal with your interval training, switch to the higher gear for five minutes, and then return to the initial intensity. You can do it once or more times during your training, but you do not need to do it every time.

With interval workout your workout will be more exciting and varied while it will let your body burn fat much easier. Try to incorporate as often as possible.

Chapter 6: Tighter and better defined stomach muscles

Now it's really getting down to the nitty gritty – You want to know how you can get tight stomach muscles, a stomach which is flat, toned and sexy. The fat is gone and the stomach muscles are ready for definition.

As said before, you can't expect to do a couple of sit ups and reach the desired result just like that. You have to do a variety of other things along with it. Eat right, exercise to burn fat, use methods to sculpt your stomach.

Maybe a long time ago you thought you would do as much sit ups as possible every day and you will have toned muscles, or maybe you buy one of these exercise machines for stomach muscles, you can see them all the time on TV. But it is not quite that simple.

It is very important when you train your muscles as well as during the endurance workout that you do not forget to breathe. Especially when you are exercising your muscles you are prone to hold your breath. You should not do that at all . Just breathe normal.

When you do sit ups you should exhale when you sit up and inhale when you lay down. The same principle applies when you do push-ups. You should always exhale when you are doing the difficult part of the exercise, where you use the most energy.

Try exercises where you have to remain in the same position for a couple seconds – but do not forget to breathe normal!

Your torso - and why you have to exercise the entire torso

You are working on burning fat and tone your stomach in a certain way; hence you focus on your stomach area. It does make sense. But before you even start you have to know exactly what part of your stomach you need to train. This is more than the muscles you can see right in front.

In order to get those toned stomach muscles you will have to exercise all your torso muscles, which means all the muscles around your waist. Of course stomach muscles will give you those six pack abs. But your torso muscles will be the ones who transform your simple stomach muscles into six pack abs.
If you only tone your *rectus abdominis* muscles (the one in front) and neglect the rest - you will look quite funny!

The torso muscles stabilize your torso and help to stand upright. They protect our back and our internal organs. You will look even more attractive if those muscles are in shape as well.

Torso muscles are not only muscles in the stomach area, but also in your back, your pelvic floor and your hips. There are even some torso muscles called *transversus abdominis*, which hide behind other muscles, yet they are essential for the overall result.

Bottomline is: To exercise your stomach muscles means to exercise your entire torso. A strong and in shape torso will present you with the abs of your dreams.

Why can't I just do Sit Ups?

Sit ups are a great exercise, but there are various reasons why you cannot rely on them to tone your stomach muscles

One of the most important reasons why you should not only to sit ups to tone and define your stomach is that it is easy to get stomach muscles which will look great from the front, but from the side they will appear bulky and bulgy.

The reason for this is that you are only focusing on the *rectus abdominis* muscles (the stomach muscles in the front). For a lean and toned overall picture you will have to exercise the entire muscle group in this area, inclusive of the *transversus abdominis*, the largest muscle, which carries the rectus abdominis and the rest of the torso muscles.

Simple sit ups will not train your stomach muscles the way they are meant to be, i.e. to keep your spine straight and that your movement is correct and secure. If your stomach muscles are exercised right, not only do they make sure of the correct and secure movement, but also look fabulous.

Together with exercising these groups you can do something else which will be wonderful for your body. You can use exercises beneficial for your entire body. Push-ups are perfect for exercising your waist and stomach because you are tightening your torso muscles as well.   .

This is an isometric form of training, which means that we strengthen the entire muscle group by keeping it in a fixed position for some time. Exercises like push-ups are for the entire body as they exercise arms, shoulders torso muscles and legs.

Just sit ups and push-ups is not enough, because you will only focus on a one part of your body. They are important and you should do them consistently in combination with other important exercises. This is the only way to get the abs you dream of.

So what about these abs workout machines you see advertised?

Abs workout equipment – these great new pieces of equipment you see on TV presented by super attractive smiling models making exercising seem so easy - and better yet inches and fat melt away making incredible abs appear just like that?

Fact is that these machines do train your stomach muscles. That is correct. But they do not do a bit of good for the layers of fat above the muscles. Your six pack abs will hide under the fat later on. Besides this you can achieve the same results are home without any expensive equipment.

Most people buy these machines because their presence in the living room should motivate them to exercise. Or maybe they really think that those machines work miracles and make stomach muscles appear and that they do not have to do anything to lose weight and get in shape. Unfortunately this is not the case and after some time they just collect dust.

Which exercises are great for stomach muscles?

You will be happy to hear that there are quite a lot of different options for you to choose from when it comes to exercising your stomach and torso muscles, and to strengthen you back and the entire body. And besides this you will really look sexy. Let's start with the essentials. The following are some good exercises for your torso muscles and do not require any special equipment

Tighten your stomach - this isn't actually a special exercise, but something you can do anytime and anywhere to strengthen your stomach muscles. Just tighten the muscles around your stomach area. The same way you would do it lifting something heavy to protect your back. Just do it over and over every day, this is a constant stomach muscle exercise.

Sit-ups, even though sit-ups alone won't be enough – they are still a very useful exercise to strengthen and tone your stomach muscles. Pay attention to your posture while you pull yourself up so that your back and your invertebrate neck area are protected.

Sit-ups are performed lying flat on your back, with your knees flexed, feet on the ground and your hands beside your head. Contract your stomach muscles and roll yourself up. Relax when you are lying back down. Don't pull your head up with your hands behind your head. You can also do the sit-ups by crossing your arms in front of your chest and tucking in your knee – some people like this version better.

Don't do more than 100 sit-ups during one exercise period, which does not have to be all at once. If you prefer, you can break them up to beginning, middle and of your exercises.

Push-ups – Push-ups are considered an exercise for the upper body, however they are just as well for your stomach muscles, torso, and legs. They fulfill several purposes at once.

To perform a push-up you should put your hands on the ground underneath your shoulders, your body is stretched up from head to toe, (toes are on the ground) and the stomach is tightened. Bend your elbows, lower your body until it is about 12 inches above the ground and
pull it back up.

Push-ups are not easy to do, but as you will get stronger with time you will be able to do more. In the beginning perhaps push-ups might be too difficult for you. You can start out by leaving your knees on the ground while keeping your body straight. It does not matter if you decide to do real push-ups or beginner push-ups; try to do twenty repetitions up to three times during your exercises.

Planks – Planks are a super method to get your stomach and torso muscles in shape, but you have to do them properly so they are really effective.

You are going to start out in a similar position like the push-ups, just that your elbows are on the ground instead of your hands. Lift your body off the ground so that your lower arms and your toes touch the ground. Pay attention to stretching your body and tighten your stomach muscles. Now keep this position about 20 to 45 seconds while only your elbows, lower arms, and toes touch the ground.

If you can't manage to keep this position at least 20 seconds try an easier version of planks where you leave your knees on the ground. Then work yourself up to the real plank.

Side planks – this is a good way to exercise your torso muscles as well. Lay on the ground on your side with your elbow underneath your shoulder, the lower part of your arm is flat on the ground. Your feet are either about 15 inches apart, one in front of the other, or your feet are altogether. The latter is the more difficult version. Keep your body stretched from head to toe, tighten your stomach, and try to lift yourself off the ground. Keep this position 10 seconds. Alternate between both sides of your body with three sets each.

Lunges – Lunges help to define your stomach muscles as you need to work your stomach muscles in order to keep your balance.

For a proper lunge you need to stand straight with your stomach tightened and a straight back. Just take a step to the front and bend your knee (the knee in front should not be farther out then the toes of your foot), pull yourself back up with the help of your legs. Repeat this motion several times while changing legs. Your goal should be 20 – 30 repetitions per leg.

Hip Lifts – This exercise trains your stomach muscles, your back and your buttocks.

For a hip lift you need to lie on your back, hands to your side, knees bent and feet apart as wide as your hips. Slowly lift your hips off the ground and tighten your stomach. Make sure not to bend your back and keep it straight. Keep this position very a few seconds with your stomach completely flat and lower your back down to the ground again, starting with the upper vertebrae down to your buttocks. Repeat this exercise several times. Try to accomplish 20 lifts per workout unit.

V-Sit-Ups – This is an advanced exercise for your stomach muscles, and a very effective one besides that. Even if you can only do on in the beginning, stick to it and you will improve and do more time after time.

In order to do a V-sit-up you need to sit on the floor, your arms slightly behind you with your hands flat on the ground, your fingers pointing towards your toes. Your elbows should be slightly bent. Your legs are and knees are bending, feet flat on the ground. Slowly lean back on your hands, bent your elbows and push your legs away from your body. Then lean forward and bring your legs back towards your chest, bending your knees and keep your feet above the ground. Stretch back and forth multiple times. With time you should be able to do about 100 V-sit-ups.

Squats - Squats are a great workout for your lower body and your torso muscles. They are easy to do and very effective.

In order to do a squat you need to stand upright with your feet about shoulder width apart, and your toes pointing slightly outwards. Go down as if you wanted to sit down in a chair, buttocks backwards. While you are "sitting" tighten your stomach muscles, stretch out your arms to the front to keep your balance , and keep your back straight while bending slightly forward (as your buttocks are in the same position as sitting down in a chair). Stand straight up. You should be able to do about 100 squats in one workout unit.

Back stretching – as the name already tells you, this is a great exercise for your back, while other torso muscles are worked as well, including your stomach muscles.

In order to stretch your back you need to lay on the ground with your face facing the floor, stretching your legs and feet. Now lift up your head, shoulders, and feet. Roll your shoulders backwards and stretch your arms on the side towards your feet. Now lift your feet, head and shoulders while you tighten your stomach muscles. Keep this position for a couple seconds, then relax. Your goal should be 10 -12 of these exercises.

Russian Twist – This exercise focuses on the muscles on your side, you are going to stretch your waist with it. Though it is an advanced exercise you will be able to do it with a little practice. At some point you should be able to do three sets with about 10 – 12 repetitions. Even if you only manage to do 8 -10 repetitions it will be great for your stomach.

For the Russian twist you need to lay flat on your mat on the floor, your knees bend with your feet on the ground.

Stretch your arms facing away from you with the palms of your hands together. Now sit upright so that your body and your legs will form a V-shape. Turn to one side and then to the other moving your waist while keeping your arms stretched out. Lay back down. This is a Russian twist.

REMARKS: Try to avoid exhausting yourself too much with these exercises. If you feel pain at any time, besides a higher heart rate, heavy breathing, and challenging of your muscles, you will need to stop while paying attention to your position. You are a beginner and should always start out with beginner positions – if there are beginner positions for the particular exercise - until you are familiar with the routine.

Just like always, if you have any questions or concerns, perhaps about old injuries which could potentially surface again with the exercises, you should ask your physician.

Exercise, tone, and define your stomach muscles in 30 minutes a day

Now you know how you will get those fabulous abs. Exercising is key just like your nutrition plays a vital part. You can exercise your torso muscles day and night, but there is no use for it if there is still this roll of fat hiding the muscles underneath it.

Eat healthy and lose weight. You can be certain that your workout for your stomach muscles will also create this incredible waist you would like to show off.

Now let's take a look at how your exercise plan to build your stomach muscles should be set up:

At first you have to incorporate stomach muscles, torso and exercises for the entire body in your program which is described in this chapter. You should do these exercises three to four times per week. If you like this could be every other day. Your muscles will be able to relax on the days in between. Those are the days where you will do endurance training.

You should be able to do a lot of stomach muscle and torso exercises in half an hour. Try to do a lot of repetitions and maybe go a little over half an hour; however, don't overdo it as you are doing the routines one after the other with little or no break in between.

If you are a beginner and are not able to do the repetitions I mentioned for every exercise, then you might take less than half an hour. In this case just take a brisk walk for the last couple of minutes, dance in your living room, or walk standing still. Just find an activity to fill the rest of half an hour.

Repeat these exercises over and over again and you will see that you are also doing a little bit of endurance exercises and burn additional fat.

This is how your stomach muscle workout could look:

Whenever you have a „stomach muscle day" you will not do any endurance training. If possible try to work out at the same time each day. This way you will not forget anything. If you are setting a time, working out will be a routine quickly. If you can't do that make sure that you write down everything in a calendar, or try any other with to remind yourself about your stomach muscle workout.

You can use a mat for working out, or just the floor – it is entirely up to you. Wear lose fitting clothes so you can move freely. You should warm up for a couple minutes , maybe dance around for 2 – 3 minutes. This way your muscles are warmed up and losened.

Now you are going to start with your exercises. You can just do the same exercises I have listed or you can create your own routine. The main point is to do everything, no matter in which order.

After working out you should stretch for a couple minutes. This way your muscles will relax easier and you will feel good.

As a beginner you might only be able to do a few repetitions for each exercise. Don't worry. Just do as many as possible, take a break and start over. Each time you are finished with an exercise you should be exhausted. You do not have to take it to the extreme of complete exhaustion until something is starting to hurt. It is enough that you feel you have worked out the muscle group well enough.

If you want to show of your great muscles later on you need to stick to exercising your stomach muscles three to four times a week, and that for the entire half an hour. If you can do that you will see the results very soon. While you are losing weight and burn fat with you work out and healthy eating habits your stomach muscles will start to show.

You can always intensify your work out by using dumbbells for certain exercises, like lunges and squats, if your stomach exercises will seem too easy at some point. You can intensify your sit ups by putting a weight behind your head or over your chest.

You should switch the sequence of your routine so that you r muscles won't know ahead of time what is coming up next. This is actually very important as working out is not very effective if you do not switch up your routine.

If you like, you can do more intense work outs on certain days. Don't forget that some of the exercises have beginner and advanced positions. If you started out with the beginner exercise you can switch to the advanced exercise after some time.

This is an example for a work out plan in order to bring your abs in top form:

1st Week:
Sunday: Sit-Ups, Push-ups, Planks, Side Planks, Hip Lifts, V-Sit-Ups, Back stretching, Russian Twist, Lunges, Squats
Tuesday: Squats (more intense with light weights), Planks, Push-ups, Side Planks, Back stretching, Lunges (more intense with light weights), Russian Twist, V-Sit-Ups, Push-ups, Sit-Ups (more intense with light weights)
Thursday: Sit-Ups, Push-ups, Planks, Side Planks, Hip Lifts, V-Sit-Ups, Back stretching, Russian Twist, Lunges, Squats
Saturday: Squats (more intense with light weights), Planks, Push-ups, Side Planks, Back stretching, Lunges (more intense with light weights), Russian Twist, V-Sit-Ups, Push-ups, Sit-Ups (more intense with light weights)

2nd Week:
Monday: Sit-Ups, Push-ups, Planks, Side Planks, Hip Lifts, V-Sit-Ups, Back stretching, Russian Twist, Lunges, Squats
Wednesday: Squats (more intense with light weights), Planks, Push-ups, Side Planks, Back stretching, Lunges (more intense with light weights), Russian Twist, V-Sit-Ups, Push-ups, Sit-Ups (more intense with light weights)
Friday: Sit-Ups, Push-ups, Planks, Side Planks, Hip Lifts, V-Sit-Ups, Back stretching, Russian Twist, Lunges, Squats

Stick to a workout routine like this for your stomach and torso muscles. You can be sure that you have done everything that is necessary in just half an hour.

On the days where you won't work out your stomach muscles you will do the endurance workout in order to burn fat.

Aides for stomach muscle workout

You can do all the exercises we described in this chapter without any special equipment. They work well and you will see success very soon. This is great for those of us who do not want to or cannot afford to buy expensive equipment.

Following some tips if you should be interested in some aides for your exercise routines:

Weights – I briefly mentioned this before. Light dumbbells (1 to 3 pounds) can be bought pretty cheap. You can intensify your workout and it can make quite a difference despite the dumbbells being rather light. If you do not want to spend any money you can just use some cans with vegetables, soup as weights instead. You can also use a light fitness ball .

Matt – For those of you who do not like to lie on the floor I would recommend a sports or yoga mat. Those mats have a slightly sticky surface, which will help to make your movements more solid and you will not slip.

Gymnastic ball – a gymnastic ball for sit ups, Push-ups, and back stretching. If you are using a gymnastic ball the exercise will be more difficult and intense. You should take your time and learn how to use the gymnastic ball if you are just starting out. Gymnastikball - Viele Leute verwenden Gymnastikbälle für Sit-Ups, Push-ups und Backstretching. Mit einem Gymnastikball wird die Übung intensiver und schwieriger. Fangen Sie gerade erst an, dann lassen Sie sich Zeit, bevor Sie mit dem Gymnastikball umzugehen lernen.

Don't forget about your work out diary. I already suggested it when talking about the motivation tool chest. You should log your exercise routine as well as your progress in the diary. It is an essential tool in order to keep you motivated and document your progress, and to see it written down. Vergessen Sie auch nicht auf Ihr Trainingstagebuch. Ich habe Ihnen das ja schon für Ihre Motivationswerkzeugkiste vorgeschlagen. Sie sollten Ihr Trainingsprogramm und Ihre Fortschritte in diesem Tagebuch festhalten Es ist ein ganz wichtiges Hilfsmittel, um sich zu motivieren, um die Fortschritte auch schwarz auf weiß zu sehen, die Sie gemacht haben.

A fitness room at home

There is one last thing I would like to point out with regards to your stomach muscle and torso work out, as well as your endurance work out: for any kind of exercise you are going to do at home, no matter whether it is your stomach or torso work out or an aerobic CD for your endurance training – you need a designated fitness area. Eine letzte Sache, auf die ich Sie für Ihr Bauchmuskel und Rumpfworkoutund Ihr Ausdauerworkouthinweisen will: für jede Art von Übung, die Sie zuhause machen wollen, ob das nun Ihrer Bauchmuskel- und Rumpfübungen oder eine Aerobic-DVD für Ihr Ausdauerworkoutsind, Sie brauchen einen Fitnessbereich.

No reason to panic! I know most of us do not have an extra room at home which can be used for exercising only. Most of us work out in the living room, or even the bedroom. This is absolutely ok, and there is nothing bad about it.

Nonetheless you have to make enough space to move and make the best of your exercises. It may be a space which you are setting up temporary and take down each time you finish, or a dedicated space. It is all depending on how much space you do have available.

The most ideal solution is if you are one of the fortunate people who are able to set up a fitness room in your house.

For your fitness room or area you just need a simple space, which is big enough to move freely and store the things you need to use for an effective workout.

Some people love to watch TV; others like to listen to music while they work out. In this instance you will need a TV or stereo system close by. Others again like to have a quiet and private space. In this case your bedroom may be more suitable. Or you manage to schedule your work out when no one else is at home and can't disturb you.

Your personal fitness room can be the place where you store all your DVD's, weights, mats and other training items. This way you can access them quickly. You should also keep some clean towels handy to wipe yourself off as soon as you are starting to sweat.

The area where you work out should be pleasant and clean. Your surrounding does have either a positive or negative influence on your mood and motivation. Who would like to work out in a place where it is messy and chaotic? You would think about the mess during the entire work out, which you will have to clean up after you are finished! If you are a messy person by nature you may not have enough space to move about freely. As you can see it is very important to have a clean and neat space.

It is quite possible that it is easier for you to exercise without anyone disturbing you. It would be best if you have a private space for your work out. If this is not the case you can schedule to exercise before everyone else will get up in the morning, or when your children are in school, take a nap, or when your partner is not at home, maybe because he is walking the dog.

Chapter 7: Final Results and maintenance

You read this e-book and are burning to finally start to lose weight and build muscle – just do it! If you already started out , continue to do it!

Your goal is a healthier, slimmer, and toned body, with a flat stomach and abs. You would like to achieve the self-confidence of someone who knows how good he looks. Depending on the fitness level and weight you are starting out with this may take months to reach your goal. Don't let anything stand in your way. If you never start you will never reach your goal.

Experts will tell you that it is best to combine losing weight and working out, with the aim on losing about 1 to 2 pounds a week. It does not sound like much, and if you are going to eat a lot less and work out a lot, you could potentially accomplish more than this. Even though this is right, you should always lose weight in a reasonable timeframe – a timeframe which feels good for your body and which will keep you healthy. You will be able to maintain your weight much better if you are losing it slow, steady, and the right way and not if you are losing it super-fast.

Why should you trouble yourself to lose weight and exercise your stomach muscles as well as the rest of your body, if you cannot maintain your weight afterwards?

Your final result will never be the same as everyone else's. You have to keep in mind, that no matter how much you work out and lose weight, chances are you will not look like your favorite celebrity. Celebrities have an advantage we do not have on pictures – and it is called photo shopping.

As I have already mentioned previously, a female would not be able to eat more than 900 calories in order to achieve a weight like most of the female celebrities have. And that is just not healthy, no matter what Hollywood will tell you!

Whether you are male or female, the final result is depending on your bodies' constitution, and what you have invested in your weight and fitness.

In any case, you can lose weight and burn fat. You can get stomach muscles to be proud of, and even show them off on the beach. You can reach the point where you love your body, feel more confident and are 100% ready to face the world.

How you maintain what you accomplished

You lost weight and now have a nice flat stomach with well-defined muscles. As an added bonus you can see that the rest of your body looks good as well. Now it is about time to maintain those looks.

For some people maintaining their weight and keep the muscle is just as frightening as the actual weight loss and work out. But it is relatively easy to preserve your body just the way it turned out to be. Just like with losing weight and working out it requires discipline and dedication, but it will also pay off in the long run.

The first step it to keep eating healthy. This means to eat with your health in the back of your mind, and keep working out every day.

To keep the same diet plan as losing weight is a good start. You do not have to lose any more weight and can add a few calories. But always keep in mind, in order to keep a flat stomach you will still need to keep your fat intake regulated.

We already discussed fat in general. You need certain fats in your nutrition so that your body can function properly and you stay healthy. This is quite alright, just keep eating the right kind of fat and stay away from the wrong ones, just as if they were big hairy spiders or even brain eating zombies.

We also discussed all the other food groups. Healthy beverages and why it is so important to keep a good balance in what you eat. This is the base for a healthy eating habit which will keep your body trim and toned.

Does this mean you will never be able to eat another piece of birthday cake or a bowl of chips? No. It is just about a tradeoff. You will exchange your big piece of cake for a beautiful flat stomach. Instead take a small piece of cake and just a handful of chips.

Pay attention to healthy nutrition. This is a big part of the way leading you to your desired goal and will keep you there

Besides healthy foods you need to keep working out. And that means every day. If you want to have a flat stomach you have to sign up for the program. To sacrifice half an hour every day of your life sounds very reasonable, doesn't it?

Continue with the program you have established to get in shape, which means endurance training, strength training, stretching and weight training. If you notice that you are not staying in shape the way you want to, you need to intensify your workout routine.

People who keep their body in shape work out every day.

Besides focusing on your stomach muscles you need to keep in mind that you can work on being in shape in many different ways. Work out your stomach muscles, but do not neglect the rest of your body. To lose weight and be toned can only be accomplished if you are working on all your muscle groups and tone your entire body.

To keep a trim and toned body also means to get used to eating healthy. This way you will feel great , be resilient against getting sick, and look fabulous.

Your work out sessions

We talked about the necessity to keep your work out stimulating while you are working on getting in shape. The same is true for maintaining your shape. Your body as well as your soul needs to remain interested and motivated – not bored and disinterested. .

Pay attention to the advice for keeping your exercising routine challenging, as we already discussed before. This will guaranteed that all your muscle groups will stay in great shape. Achten Sie darauf, sich an die Anleitungen für abwechslungsreiches Workoutzu halten, die wir vorher schon besprochen haben. So bleiben Ihre Muskelgruppen in guter Form.

- Establish a balanced work out plan with enough changes to keep your body and soul challenged.
- When you are working on endurance change your distance, pace, and intensity routine.
- With strengthening exercises, either with or without weights, pay attention to keep some routines more intense than others.

What to do when you feel weak or are tempted to be lazy and eat wrong

It is unavoidable that this will happen at some point. There will be the day when you eat that piece of cake and will not work out, because you simply do not care. That you will skip the point everyone else reaches sooner or later is not credible. We are all just human beings – and we are going to be tempted to do things sometimes, which are not really good for us.

My advice for such moments:

First, do not lie to yourself. Don't think you will never be tempted to eat too much, to eat the wrong things, to slouch on the couch and rather watch TV than to work out.

Instead be aware that this will happen and you will have a plan in place to resist the temptation.

If you feel this moment approaching, get your motivation tool chest. Or better yet place your motivation tools where you cannot avoid seeing them on the way to the piece of cake or to the TV.

Look at your collection. Photos from before and after the program. Your diary. Your list with proverbs and quotes. The label of the size of your pants when you were much heavier and the one you wear now. Everything you went through to reach your goal. Your goal is still to stay healthy, trim and toned – and not to wharf down bags of chips while you sit on the porch.

But what will happen if you cannot resist this temptation?

First of all you should not feel guilty and not suffer more than necessary. Ok, so you made a mistake. Have a conversation with yourself and try to understand why this has happened.

And then you have to get back on the right path. Forgive yourself and stop torturing yourself with guilt. Just give yourself a fresh start. You can still work out today. You can still find options to cut some calories tomorrow, to trim some fat from your meals in order to repair some of the damage you did today. (Just do not exaggerate, after all everything needs to remain healthy above all).

Put an entry in your diary if this helps. Maybe you really had a rough day at work and thought you would feel better after eating a quart of ice cream. Was this really the reason? Try to track the instances which make you react in a problematic way. It will help you to deal with them better in the future.

The motivation tool chest

We talked about it several times already, but it is well worth it to talk about it again. Most of us have to be constantly reminded why we are doing what we are doing, and for each of us some things will work better than others.

Consider the following for your motivation tool chest:

- Photos of yourself before you started to work out and lose weight, photos of your progress, and photos of the moment when you reached your goal.
- An eating and exercising diary.
- A diary for your experiences, feelings and moods.
- A list of people you can turn to whenever you need some help or encouraging words.
- A list of proverbs and quotes, which will help you to feel strong, self-confident and able to feel your emotions.
- Rewards

What you should avoid from now on

Your new body demands that you will avoid certain things for the rest of your life. We already discussed how you can resist temptation to eat wrong, a) it is unhealthy, and b) it will lead you to putting on weight. This is a basic law to maintain your weight.

We also discussed the fact that you have to avoid to be lazy when it comes to your work our routine. You will have to exercise every day for the rest of your life. (In exceptional times you can be without one day of working out, or when you are sick).

But what else should you avoid?

It is very important to stay away from people who can influence your progress in a negative way. This may sound harsh, as most of the time it will be family and friends telling you "C'mon that second helping of Lasagna won't hurt you."

If you cave in every time when someone tries to make you eat, drink, or adapt to their habits the same way they do, it will really cause serious damage to maintaining your new trim body.

Keep in mind that perhaps you need to spend less time with certain people who may encourage you to fall back into your old and unhealthy habits in order to maintain a healthier lifestyle, which of course does not mean to cut these people out of your life completely.

Another species you should try to avoid (or with whom you should at least associate less) are the people who bring you down. People, who eat too much, are lazy and self-sufficient, but behind your back they will envy you about your new lifestyle and success.

Surround yourself with people who are understanding and encouraging, and will not tempt you to life „ poorly" (even you are conscious about it or not).

If you had places like restaurants, pubs, bars, etc., you did like to visit before, or habits where you ate things which are not good for you, then you will have to avoid them and find new places, where you don't have to rely that much on your determination to resist the temptation.

I know, this section sounds like you were a drug addict who is trying to avoid falling back into his old, bad habits. In a certain way this is exactly what can happen to you. Old habits, like eating too much and the wrong food, and being lazy will make you dependent and are really damaging to yourself.

You are just in the process to develop new, healthy habits, and a healthy, trim body. You will have to continue to live to preserve this healthy and good looking body from now on.

What if you put on weight?

Your weight will always fluctuate up and down. If you put on four pounds and lose it again right away, that's ok. Not a big deal. But if you put on 4 pounds, and another 4 pounds, and then another pound it creates a big problem. Put an end to it before things spiral out of control.

There are several things you need to do if you put on too much weight:

- Immediately get back to your diet plan – the one you had when you are started to lose weight. You have to be very persistent. Figure out when you are eating too much – and put a stop to it!
- Intensify your work out. If you are working out half an hour now, add another 15 minutes. Or work out harder during the half hour.
- Get your motivation tool chest and use it.
- Get some help. If you are part of a work out group, of if you started to lose weight together with friends, sound the alarm and get encouragement and motivation from them.
- If you still keep putting on weight and all your efforts to get this situation under control you need to consult a physician and exclude any health problems.

What if you get sick or injured?

It will happen. You are in the middle of losing weight and are diligently exercising every day, maintain your weight, and all of a sudden you are getting sick, catch a cold, twist your ankle or pull a muscle.

The good thing is that you became much healthier by eating right and working out, and the risk of getting sick or injured has decreased. Your immune system is much stronger and better able to protect yourself from injuries. Still you can get sick or injured.

So what are you going to do if this happens?

You are sick, for example having a cold. It is best if you will let your body rest and allow healing itself. It is unreasonable to exercise in this situation. Your body will need its energy to fight the virus brewing inside of you.

You should still pay attention to eat well, as this will aide your immune system and help to win the battle much quicker.

As soon as you are free of fever and feel up to it , try to go for a walk , swim , or ride your bike – but do not overdo it as your body still needs energy for recuperating. The better you feel, the sooner you can step up your exercise plan.

If you are getting seriously ill and need to be treated by a physician you should discuss with him when and in how much you can start working out again.

If you have been injured you need to pay special attention in order not to escalate the injury of a certain area. Often it is enough to just change your workout routine until the injury is healed completely.

Likewise, if your injury is so serious that is needs to be treated by a physician, you need to consult him about starting to work out.

Of course it is frustrating to stop your work out due to illness or injury. But it would be much worse if you would start to exercise again before your body is ready for a stress.
Continue with your healthy diet plan and only do what you really are able to.

Give advice to others to stay fit yourself

Sometimes the best way to help yourself is to help others. This proves to be true especially when you are trying to lose weight or work out. If you have gone through a certain situation it is easier to identify yourself with the problems others may face as well in the same situation.

If you have been successful and lost weight permanently and built a toned body with abs anyone would like to have, then you are destined to help others who are just at the beginning of their journey.

I am not trying to tell you that you should mutate into a city wide known fitness expert, or health and nutrition counselor. Encourage people, go work out with them together if there is an opportunity. I am trying to encourage you to help other reach their goals, give them helpful tips whenever you can. This is another way to affirm and remind yourself about all the things you have to pay attention to in order to keep trim and toned.

To help others will at the same time help you to be responsible for your own actions. You can't advise others to exercise more if you won't do it as well. You cannot give them tips about healthy eating, how you lose weight the right way if you won't eat healthy yourself to lose weight or maintain your weight after you lost weight.

This is a very efficient way for you to stay on course.

The program I introduced is not a miracle diet, or a miracle combination of exercises after which you will look like a celebrity.

It is much more a common sense program. If you stick to it you will see results pretty soon. Great results!

You can achieve amazing abs and a toned body with only half an hour of exercising every day, this is absolutely possible. But you have to show dedication and commitment. You have to eat healthy – the right meals with the right serving sizes. This is the only way it will be successful.

Yes, you can burn fat and build muscle in just half an hour per day! You can get this beautiful body, more self-confidence, and yes, even better chances on the job market, on dates, and in your relationship. You will be healthier and have a much better immune system.

Just believe in yourself!

It will be worth the time and effort you are going to invest! To invest in health and self-confidence, to invest in yourself, this is the best investment in your future!

Good luck and success,

Yours cordially,
Jörg Weber
http://www.welchediaet.de

P.S.
I hope this e-book provided you with some great tips and tricks how you can live healthier and longer. If you have learned anything from it and can apply it for your own

success, I would appreciate if you would leave a positive feedback for me.
Following is the link:
http://www.amazon.com/Burning-Belly-Truth-about-ebook/dp/B007GPT404/

If you are unhappy, please do not hesitate to let me know by email (info@welchediaet.de), so I can improve this book. Please also keep in mind that you will receive future editions completely free of charge. Just talk to customer service. Perhaps your comments and suggestions will already be included in the next book.

I hope you will have great six pack abs!
Yours,
Jörg Weber

Did you read my second book?
http://www.amazon.com/develop-Abdominal-Muscles-Training-ebook/dp/B007R4E9JK

Table of Content

Introduction

Chapter 1: Why a flat Stomach and a toned Figure are better for the body

Chapter 2: The fairytale about cutting fat and a flat stomach

Chapter 3: Healthy Eating

Chapter 4: Losing Weight

Chapter 5: Burning Fat

Chapter 6: Tighter and better defined stomach muscles

Chapter 7: Final Results and maintenance

Made in the USA
Lexington, KY
07 July 2012